FLAT STOMACH AFTER PREGNANCY COOKBOOK

Dr. Penny Watson

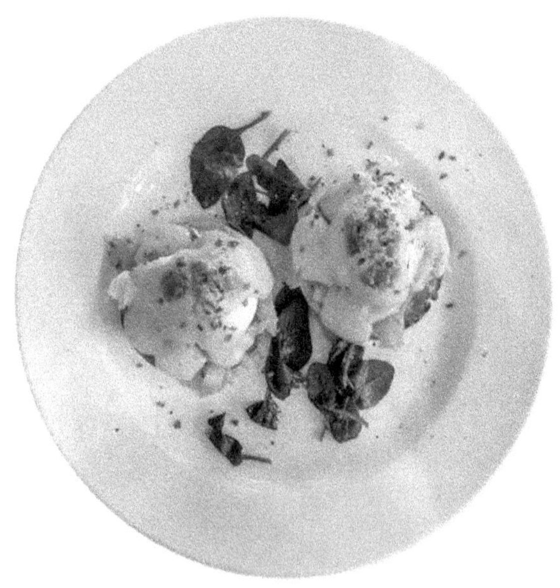

TABLE OF CONTENT

INTRODUCTION

Achieving a flat stomach after pregnancy is a common goal for many new mothers, but it's essential to approach this goal with patience and realistic expectations. Pregnancy causes significant changes in a woman's body, and the process of recovery varies from person to person.

Here are some important considerations when aiming for a flat stomach after pregnancy:

1. Postpartum Healing Takes Time: It's crucial to understand that the body needs time to heal after childbirth, especially if you had a vaginal delivery or a cesarean section. Your uterus needs time to shrink back to its prepregnancy size, and your abdominal muscles need time to recover.

2. Focus on Core Strength: Strengthening your core muscles is essential for regaining abdominal tone. This includes the transverse abdominis, rectus abdominis, and obliques. Gentle core exercises can help, but consult with a healthcare provider or a postpartum fitness specialist before starting any specific workouts.

3. Pelvic Floor Exercises: Pelvic floor exercises, such as Kegels, are important for strengthening the muscles that support your pelvic organs and can contribute to improved core stability.

4. Balanced Nutrition: Eating a wellbalanced diet that includes plenty of fruits, vegetables, lean proteins, whole grains, and healthy fats is essential for overall health and can aid in weight management.

5. Breastfeeding: If you are breastfeeding, it can help burn extra calories and contribute to postpartum weight loss. However, it's crucial to ensure you're consuming enough calories and nutrients to support breastfeeding and your overall health

6. Hydration: Staying hydrated is essential for overall health and can help with digestion and metabolism.

7. Gradual Exercise: Start with gentle, lowimpact exercises like walking, postnatal yoga, or swimming. As you regain strength and endurance, you can gradually incorporate more intense workouts.

8. Consult a Professional: Consider working with a postnatal fitness specialist or a physical therapist who can assess your specific needs and provide tailored exercises to target your abdominal muscles safely.

9. Avoid Crash Diets: Rapid weight loss or extreme dieting is not recommended during the postpartum period, especially if you are breastfeeding. It can affect your milk supply and overall health.

10. Embrace Your Body: Remember that your body has gone through a significant transformation to bring new life into the world.

Embrace your postpregnancy body and give yourself grace. Selflove and selfacceptance are essential during this time.

11. Seek Medical Advice: If you have concerns about diastasis recti (a separation of the abdominal muscles) or other postpartum issues, consult with a healthcare provider or physical therapist for guidance and support.

12. Consistency and Patience: Achieving a flat stomach after pregnancy takes time and consistency. Stay committed to a healthy lifestyle, and remember that results may not be immediate.

Every woman's postpartum journey is unique, and it's essential to prioritize your health and wellbeing above all else. Rather than focusing solely on achieving a flat stomach, aim for a strong and functional core, good overall health, and a positive selfimage. Your body has accomplished an incredible feat, and it deserves care, respect, and appreciation.

CHAPTER ONE

Home Remedies To Get A Flat Tummy After Delivery

Admit it, mums! Getting back a flat tummy after delivery is something that every mum dreams of. Some work really hard for it, some give up altogether and others swear by Spanx to mask the extra rolls. Well, the good news is that as stubborn as they seem, those fats aren't impossible to get rid of. Here are some simple home remedies and tips for a flat tummy after pregnancy that will definitely help you.

Tips For A Flat Tummy After Pregnancy

Abdominal binding

One of the most effective tips for a flat tummy after pregnancy is to bind your tummy for as many hours as you can in a day.

Living in Singapore means that you are definitely familiar with postnatal massage and many mums find the traditional Malay bengkung wrap to be extremely effective.

Of course this is not an option for mums who have just had a csection. Professional massage therapists and doctors do not recommend such abdominal binding until at least four to six weeks have passed.

Csection mums are strongly recommended to use abdominal binders. Your doctor is likely to get you to put one on as soon as a day after your surgery. Trust me when I say that it helps! The trick is in making sure that the binder is really tight and secure. If you're worried about your incision, you can cushion it with an unused sanitary pad then use the binder over it.

Lotions

There is a myriad of topical lotions in the market that promise to help you as part of the many tips for achieving a flat tummy after pregnancy.

Especially if you're breastfeeding, do check the ingredients carefully and ensure that the cream is safe for nursing mums to use.

Look out for creams containing Collagen, Vitamins A, C and E. Massaging such creams over your tummy will improve blood flow and tighten your tummy.

If time permits, you can also use homemade lotions. One such lotion that has been proven to be effective is a hand made lotion that is a blend of 250ml of fresh grapes extract in 750ml of extra virgin oil.

Sieve the pulp before adding the grape extract to the oil.

Place the blend in a bottle and let it stay in the sun for a week.

Shake the bottle at least twice a day. Applying this homemade lotion is one of the many helpful tips for a flat tummy after pregnancy.

Ginger wraps are another favourite among mums in Singapore!

Honey Lemon

This is one of the easiest and yummiest tips for a flat tummy after pregnancy. All you got to do is to mix a glass of lukewarm water with some fresh lemon juice and half a teaspoon of honey. Drink this on an empty stomach or before meals.

If possible, drink it when you just wake up and don't drink anything else for a good half an hour before or after this.

You can also add some mint leaves and cucumber and brew the water overnight.

Cayenne pepper is not for everyone but a pinch of it goes a long way to boost your metabolism and burn that tummy fat.

Do take mint leaves in moderation though for too much of it can reduce your milk supply.

Green Tea

A cup of green tea a day keeps tummy fat away. And it's no secret that green tea is rich in antioxidants so that's an added bonus!

This makes it one of the most convenient tips for a flat tummy after pregnancy.

Do remember that you should drink green tea in moderation. Too much of it isn't good and you should limit your caffeine intake if you are breastfeeding.

And the last thing you should do is to be drinking green tea with sugar or sweeteners for that would be counter productive!

Apples

So apples don't just keep doctors away, they work well to get rid of tummy fat as well. Apples contain pectin which is helpful to burn excess tummy fat. Just like green tea, apples are rich in antioxidants and that prevents the accumulation of excess fats. Aside from it being one of the best tips for a flat tummy after pregnancy, don't forget the other many health benefits of eating apples!

A balanced diet

Remember the healthy plate model? Well, you should aim to include two portions of vegetables, a portion of fruits, whole grains, and healthy protein.

One of the most helpful tips for a flat tummy after pregnancy is to reduce your intake of salt and cut sugar out as much as you can. Avoid sodas and other carbonated drinks.

Cruciferous fruits and vegetables like papaya, mangoes, grapefruit, broccoli, and kale are great when it comes to losing abdominal fat.

As much as you want that flat tummy after pregnancy, do not compromise on the nutritional value of your food. This is essential for your recovery and even more so if you are breastfeeding.

Eat less but more frequently

Dieting is not effective and it will make you weak. Your metabolism is pretty high at this point in time so aim for two heavy meals a day and three to four small meals at regular intervals. Go heavy on breakfast.

Remember that when you eat well, you also end up burning more calories.

Sweat it out!

You are what you eat – yes, largely, but you are also how much you move (or don't move). Don't jump into HIIT training or high impact workouts shortly after giving birth. You don't want to end up with a prolapsed uterus!

Strenuous workouts are not for new mums!

Start by gradually building your endurance through walking, swimming, and cycling. Focus on cardio and when you have lost overall fat, focus on tummy toning exercises such as crunches and planks.

Mums do remember that it's impossibly to 'spot reduce' fats. You could do all the tummy exercises you want but you need cardio to get rid of overall fat.

Importantly, make sure that you do not have a diastasis recti for if you do, tummy exercises like crunches will exacerbate the problem. You need specific exercises to correct a diastasis recti.

Breastfeeding

As far as tips for a flat tummy after pregnancy go, this is of course a given.

In case you didn't already know, breastfeeding burns approximately 500 calories a day and helps your uterus to contract to its prepregnancy size. So this goes a long way in achieving a flat tummy after delivery.

H2O

Another one of the many given tips for achieving a flat tummy after pregnancy. This is cheap, extremely important and also effective.

Water rids your body of toxins and helps to reduce belly fat.

It also helps to replenish the fluids you lose so if you're breastfeeding and insanely thirsty, you need to drink a lot more water.

Added bonus – drinking more water gives you great skin!

Mums, if your confinement nanny or motherinlaw tells you that drinking water during confinement gives you a tummy you will never get rid of, please dismiss this misinformation. You need water. A lot of it!

Curry leaves and garlic

Did you know that curry leaves are great for detox? And yes, they do help you to get rid of belly fats as well! As for garlic, chewing on a couple of raw garlic cloves and then drinking lemon water can help you get your flat tummy after pregnancy. This might be a bit much for some though!

There you go mums, 11 easy and effective methods to get rid of that stubborn mummy tummy.

But please be kind to yourselves and your bodies and don't rush or stress over losing weight. Don't starve yourself or deprive your baby of important nutrients by drastically cutting calories.

Don't get too caught up in losing weight that you lose out on the most precious moments! Take it easy, follow these tips for flat tummy after pregnancy and lose the weight naturally.

Remember that losing weight too rapidly is a terrible idea for you to end up with loose and saggy skin.

You have all the time in the world to lose weight so for the time being, focus on the most important moments with your babies before they are gone too soon!

Simple Home Remedies To Really Flatten Your Belly After Pregnancy

The nine months of pregnancy pass by faster than most moms imagine. As good wishes and wellmeaning (but often unsolicited) advice starts pouring in, our days get divided among meeting relatives, attending ceremonies, clicking pictures… and EATING.

Pregnancy is the time when you are allowed to – even recommended to – eat all the yummy things your heart desires. Moms will gorge on lipsmacking food only too willingly. It is only after delivery that we realise that all the weight we put on is now going to be a huge fight to shed.

After you have put your baby down for his afternoon siesta, and all other things in the house have been taken care of, you will finally have a moment to yourself.

In that moment you might find yourself standing in front of the mirror and looking at your belly, remembering those past nine months.

As those nostalgic moments end, you are left wondering if you will get rid of all that postdelivery belly fat! Most of us are left with tummy fat postpregnancy, because of the weight gain during pregnancy, and the sagged skin after delivery.

Some people tell us – "This is a permanent side effect of becoming a mother. Live with it." Do you think it is true?

No! The good news is that nothing is terminal in life… not even your postpregnancy belly fat! Here are 14 simple home remedies to reduce belly fat after delivery. We can vouch for their effectiveness, as fellow moms have tried them out!

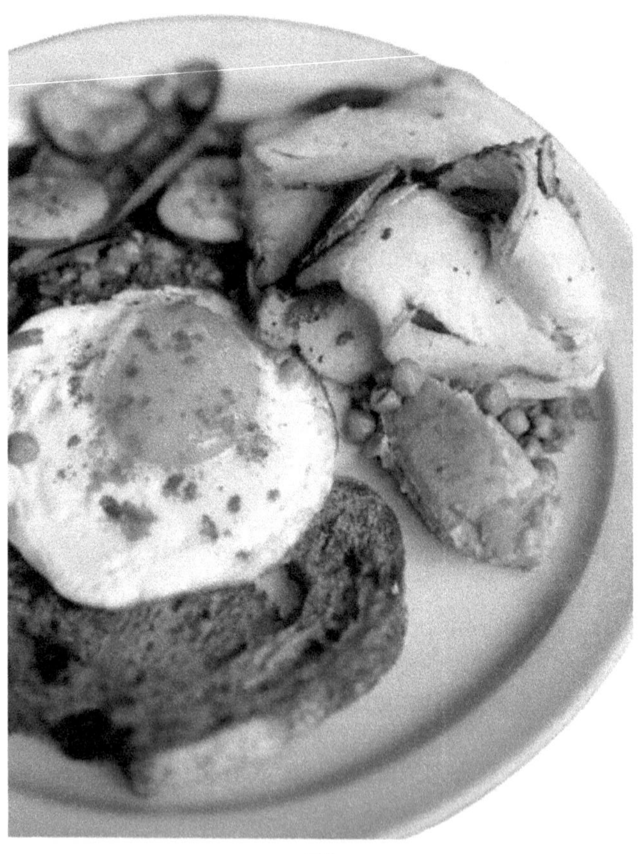

CHAPTER TWO

Home Remedies for Flat Belly After Delivery/ Pregnancy

Before you scroll down to check out the home remedies for belly fat, here is one important word of caution:

Many women around you might complain that they have 'been there, done all that' but to no avail. But do you know the single biggest mistake we make when we are trying to lose weight? We give up too soon!

For these home remedies to show the powerful results they are capable of, you have to do this: Pick any 4 of the below remedies—2 food and 2 drink recipes—continue them for at least 3 months.

When it comes to getting back in your pre pregnancy clothes, remember, consistency is the name of the game. Do not give up!

FOOD

Apple Cinnamon Oats

This is a quick fix breakfast you can have every day that is bound to make you drop pounds real fast.

It is one of the easiest home remedies to reduce tummy fat.

Take about 6 to 7 tablespoons of oats, 1 cup of milk (or half cup milk and half cup water), and add half an apple, finely diced. Add a pinch of cinnamon. If you have a sweet tooth, you can also drizzle honey on it.

You can either cook the mixture or leave it in the fridge overnight. Either way, it tastes delicious.

How it helps

Apples are rich in potassium and vitamins. Cinnamon is a great natural fatburner and oats are high on fibre. This breakfast will keep you full for longer.

Berries and Yoghurt

Whip yoghurt in a bowl. Add cut fresh berries like strawberries, blackberries, and raspberries.

To get a more consistent, even texture, you can also blend the mixture.

How it helps

Berries are loaded with vitamins and fibre. Yoghurt, on the other hand, has a good dose of proteins.

Make sure you pick a lowfat variant of yoghurt or Greek yoghurt to make sure you cut down on extra calories.

Avocado

Make this fruit your new best friend! Avocado should be your goto fruit if you are trying to lose weight.

You can add avocado to salads; you can make avocado soup, avocado milkshake, and even avocado smoothies.

How it helps

Avocado is a fruit that is rich in MUFA—monounsaturated fatty acids. These are good fats that have high satiety value and keep your snacking urges at bay.

Eggs

There are umpteen ways to have eggs—hardboiled, sunny side up, poached, omelettes, etc.

How it helps

The protein content of eggs makes it a perfect choice for losing weight and burning fat. Include at least 2 to 3 eggs in your daily diet.

Beans

Beans are another excellent choice to include proteins in your diet. They are also rich in iron. For a nutritious and fresh breakfast, you can make bean salad.

How it helps

Being high in protein and iron, beans will make you drop pounds faster. The fibre content of beans is also good to keep you feeling full at least through 3 to 4 hours.

Cayenne Pepper (Laal Mirch)

Cayenne pepper, which is one of the most effective home remedies for flat belly, can also make for a good chutney or dip. Blend finely chopped cayenne pepper, ginger, garlic, and black pepper together. Add salt to it.

You may also squeeze half a lemon into the mixture if it is too spicy or hot for you. Additionally, you may add some sugar. Have this chutney with Indian breads, like chapati, bhakari, paratha, etc.

How It Helps

Cayenne pepper helps burn fat from problem areas in the body real fast.

Garlic

Garlic can be added to most Indian recipes. You can even sauté squarediced vegetables in a little bit of olive oil and 810 garlic cloves.

For best results, let the garlic sit for 1015 minutes after chopping/crushing, before adding it to the recipe.

How it helps

Studies indicate that raw or roasted garlic helps in diabetes. It also helps in weight loss. Garlic is an excellent fatburner and will make you drop a size in about a month's time with regular consumption.

Hot Water with Honey and Lemon

If you are looking for one solid answer to the question 'how to lose belly fat at home', this is it. Generations of women will swear by the benefits of this yummy potion.

To make this drink, bring water to a boil and add a spoonful of honey; squeeze juice of half a lemon and allow it to simmer for 5 minutes. Pour into a glass and consume warm.

How it helps

This potion is one of the most potent home remedies for weight loss after pregnancy. On top of that, this drink has more than just weightloss benefits. It also acts as a blood purifier and is good for skin and complexion too!

Ginger Cardamom Mint Tea

Bring water to a boil. Add crushed fresh mint leaves, grated ginger, and 23 cardamom pods; boil it for a couple of minutes; turn off the flame and cover the vessel with a plate.

Let it stand for 5 minutes; pour in a cup and drink warm. You can even chill the mixture and have it as icetca. Also, check out this slight variation of the Ginger Flavoured Tea — perfect for rainy days!

How it helps

Each of the ingredients in the above recipe is known to have medicinal benefits. Along with that, they also help in boosting metabolism and cleansing your digestive system, which improves food absorption and helps in weight loss.

Cucumber Watermelon Juice

Dice 1 cucumber in a bowl. Add about 7 to 8 big cubes of watermelon to it. Blend the mixture together. Consume this drink without straining the juice to retain all the good fibres.

How it helps

Cucumber and watermelon are high in their water content. Moreover, watermelon also has a good amount of vitamin C. A juice made of these two fruits is a great betweenmeals drink to keep you hydrated and full.

Green Tea

Green tea is not something you will like right away. One needs to develop a taste for green tea—and it can happen.

The best idea is to buy small sachets of each of the different brands in the market, and find out which you like the most. Green tea can be made more potent by adding ingredients like cardamom, lemon, honey, cinnamon, ginger, etc.

How it helps

Green tea is not only a good fatburner, it also detoxifies your system, thereby improving digestion.

It is full of antioxidants and contains caffeine which helps in weight loss.

Celery Parsley Juice (Ajwain and Ajamod)

Blend celery and parsley together, and you will have a potent drink that will help you lose weight.

Drinking this juice in summers will also keep you cool. Celery can also be consumed raw.

How it helps

Celery is less in calories; it is a very light food. Parsley is good for kidneys.

Together, they will help you burn off the stubborn tummy fat in no time.

Bananas Almond Shake

Bananas and almonds make a really good combination. Banana almond shake is one of the most delicious home remedies for reducing belly fat after delivery. This milkshake tastes better than most foods recommended for weight loss! However, make sure you have this only about 3 times a week. To cut down on the calories of this recipe, you can use soy milk instead of regular cow's milk.

How it helps

Bananas are perhaps the yummiest source of potassium for the body. Almonds, on the other hand, provide the body with vitamin E and are a good source of essential fatty acids. All these nutrients have a high satiating value, curbing your urge to snack between meals.

WATER

How it helps

Did you know that the symptoms of hunger and thirst are the same? You may be familiar with the way your tummy grumbles when you are hungry, but do you know it also grumbles when you are thirsty?

Next time you feel 'hungry', have a glass of water and wait for about half an hour. You will notice that your 'hunger' has disappeared.

Drinking plenty of water is one of the home remedies for a flat tummy that can actually start showing results within a week. The more water you drink, the less water your body retains! What does this tell you? – Many of us misinterpret the body's signal, and end up eating more than the body needs!

Make sure you drink at least 3.54 litres of water every day. Do not drink it all at once. Have a glass of water every couple of hours.

Also, have a glass of water half an hour before your meal time – it will control your portion sizes.

So, moms, ready to get started on your weight loss and fitness journey through food and drinks? We sure are! Do let us know which of these home remedies for reducing belly fat after delivery you are going to try, and how your experience turns out.

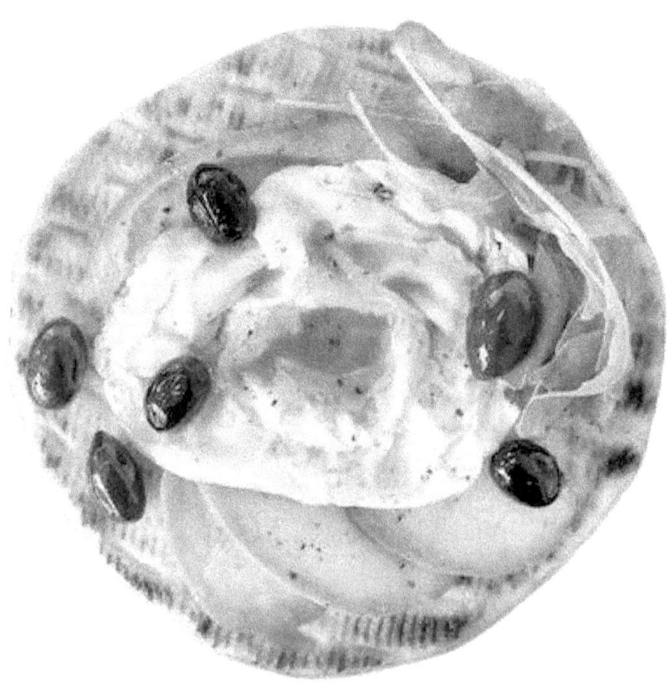

CHAPTER THREE

14 Day Meal Plan to Help Lose Belly Fat

This 30day meal plan is full of healthy recipes to help you lose weight and lose belly fat.

Trimming inches off your midsection does more than just make you feel good in your skin. Lowering belly fat, also called visceral fat, can have some serious health benefits. Excess belly fat increases risk of type 2 diabetes, heart disease and even some cancers.

The good news is that losing weight to reduce overall body fat can help, and research shows that certain foods, like chickpeas and artichokes, can be particularly helpful in trimming your waistline.

Our EatingWell approach to the flatbelly diet is a healthy one that doesn't leave you feeling deprived and hungry but rather satisfied and energized.

In addition, to those research backed flatbelly foods, this plan includes plenty of fiber and probiotic foods, like kefir and yogurt, that nourish your gut and help the good bacteria thrive. Filling up on fatburning and guthealthy foods is just one piece of the puzzle—getting plenty of exercise and adequate sleep and reducing stress all play a role in trimming belly fat.

To help with weight loss, we set this plan at 1,200 calories per day to promote a healthy weight loss of 1 to 2 pounds per week, and provide modifications to bump it up to 1,500 and 2,000calorie days, depending on your calorie needs.

Not sure you want to commit to a full 30 days? Pick and choose a few days to test out or try our shorter 7day flat belly meal plan to help you get started. And don't miss our fall and winter flatbelly plans that highlight delicious seasonal foods that fight belly fat!

FlatBelly Foods List

Fill up on these foods that research has shown can help trim your waistline and improve your gut health:

- Green tea
- Raspberries and other berries
- Artichokes
- Kimchi
- Nuts and seeds, particularly peanuts
- Kombuch
- Avocado
- Whole grains, like oats and quinoa
- Highfiber fruits and vegetables, like raspberries, apples, pears and sweet potatoes
- Lentils
- Beans, especially chickpeas
- Asparagus
- Apples
- Yogurt
- Kefir

How to MealPrep Your Week of Meals
Week 1

1. Prepare 2 servings of AppleCinnamon Overnight Oats to have for breakfast on Days 2 and 3.
2. Mealprep the Vegan Superfood Buddha Bowls to have for lunch on Days 2 through 5.
3. Prepare the Citrus Vinaigrette to have throughout the week.
4. Assemble the SlowCooker Creamy Lentil Soup Freezer Pack through Step 1 to have in Week 3.

Day 1

Breakfast (245 calories)

- 1 serving BlueberryCranberry Smoothie

A.M. Snack (62 calories)

- 1 medium orange

Lunch (325 calories)

- 1 serving Green Salad with Edamame & Beet

P.M. Snack (116 calories)

- 1 large apple

Dinner (447 calories)

- 1 serving Roasted Salmon with Smoky Chickpeas & Greens

Daily Totals: 1,194 calories, 70 g protein, 145 g carbohydrate, 34 g fiber, 39 g fat, 1,244 mg sodium

To make it 1,500 calories: Add 1 clementine to breakfast and add 1/3 cup unsalted almonds to A.M. snack.

To make it 2,000 calories: Include all modifications for the 1,500calorie day, plus add 1 serving Everything Bagel Avocado Toast to lunch and add 3 Tbsp. natural peanut butter to P.M. snack.

Day 2

Breakfast (250 calories)

- 1 serving AppleCinnamon Overnight Oats
- 1 clementine

A.M. Snack (30 calories)

- 1 plum

Lunch (381 calories)

- 1 serving Vegan Superfood Buddha Bowls

P.M. Snack (155 calories)

- 2 hardboiled eggs topped with a pinch each of salt &
  pepper

Dinner (407 calories)

- 1 serving Taco Stuffed Avocados
- 2 cups mixed greens tossed with 1 Tbsp. Citrus
  Vinaigrette

Daily Totals: 1,224 calories, 53 g protein, 121 g carbohydrate,

33 g fiber, 65 g fat, 1,150 mg sodium

To make it 1,500 calories: Add 1/3 cup unsalted dryroasted

almonds to A.M. snack.

To make it 2,000 calories: Include the modification for the

1,500calorie day, plus add 1 slice wholewheat toast with 1

Tbsp. natural peanut butter to breakfast, add 1 cup lowfat plain

Greek yogurt to A.M. snack, and add 1/4 cup guacamole with

1 bell pepper, sliced, to P.M. snack.

Day 3

Breakfast (250 calories)

- 1 serving AppleCinnamon Overnight Oats
- 1 clementine

A.M. Snack (93 calories)

- 1 cup lowfat plain kefir

Lunch (381 calories)

- 1 serving Vegan Superfood Buddha Bowls

P.M. Snack (87 calories)

- 1/2 cup nonfat plain Greek yogurt topped with 1/4 cup blueberries

Dinner (405 calories)

- 1 serving Chickpea & Potato Curry
- 2 cups mixed greens topped with 1 Tbsp. Citrus Vinaigrette

Daily Totals: 1,216 calories, 54 g protein, 163 g carbohydrate, 33 g fiber, 45 g fat, 1,194 mg sodium

To make it 1,500 calories: Add 1/3 cup walnut halves and 1 small apple to A.M. snack.

To make it 2,000 calories: Include all modifications for the 1,500calorie day, plus add 1 slice wholewheat toast with 1 Tbsp. natural peanut butter to breakfast, and add 1/4 cup almonds and increase to 1 1/4 cups yogurt at P.M. snack.

Day 4

Breakfast (245 calories)

- 1 serving BlueberryCranberry Smoothie

A.M. Snack (35 calories)

- 1 clementine

Lunch (381 calories)

- 1 serving Vegan Superfood Buddha Bowls

P.M. Snack (101 calories)

- 1 medium pear

Dinner (441 calories)

- 1 serving Buffalo Chicken Stuffed Spaghetti Squash

Daily Totals: 1,203 calories, 73 g protein, 157 g carbohydrate, 33 g fiber, 38 g fat, 935 mg sodium

MealPrep Tip: Assemble ingredients for SlowCooker Turkey Chili with Butternut Squash. Tomorrow morning, set the slow cooker to Low and cook for 8 hours so it's ready in time for dinner.

To make it 1,500 calories: Add 1/3 cup unsalted almonds to A.M. snack.

To make it 2,000 calories: Add 2 slices wholewheat toast with 2 Tbsp. natural peanut butter to breakfast and add 1/4 cup hummus with 3 medium carrots to P.M. snack.

Day 5

Breakfast (253 calories)

- 1 cup lowfat plain Greek yogurt topped with 1/4 cup raspberries and 1 1/2 Tbsp. chopped walnuts

A.M. Snack (16 calories)

- 1 cup sliced cucumber tossed with a pinch each of salt & pepper

Lunch (381 calories)

- 1 serving Vegan Superfood Buddha Bowls

P.M. Snack (35 calories)

- 1 clementine

Dinner (521 calories)

- 1 serving SlowCooker Turkey Chili with Butternut Squash
- 1 serving Guacamole Chopped Salad

Daily Totals: 1,206 calories, 68 g protein, 118 g carbohydrate, 39 g fiber, 59 g fat, 1,335 mg sodium

MealPrep Tip: Reserve 2 servings SlowCooker Turkey Chili with Butternut Squash to have for lunch on days 6 and 7.

To make it 1,500 calories: Add 1/3 cup unsalted almonds to P.M. snack.

To make it 2,000 calories: Include the modification for the 1,500calorie day, plus increase to 1/4 cup walnuts at breakfast, add 1 serving Everything Bagel Avocado Toast to A.M. snack, and add 1 large apple to lunch.

Day 6

Breakfast (245 calories)

- 1 serving BlueberryCranberry Smoothie

A.M. Snack (164 calories)

- 1/4 cup walnut halves

Lunch (371 calories)

- 1 serving SlowCooker Turkey Chili with Butternut Squash
- 1 medium apple

P.M. Snack (62 calories)

- 1 medium orange

Dinner (378 calories)

- 1 serving Shrimp Cobb Salad with Dijon Dressing

Daily Totals: 1,218 calories, 69 g protein, 142 g carbohydrate, 36 g fiber, 49 g fat, 1,258 mg sodium

To make it 1,500 calories: Add 1/3 cup unsalted almonds to P.M. snack.

To make it 2,000 calories: Include the modification for the 1,500calorie day, plus add 2 slices wholewheat toast with 2 Tbsp. natural peanut butter to breakfast, add 1 large pear to A.M. snack, and add 1 clementine to lunch.

Day 7

Breakfast (253 calories)

- 1 cup lowfat plain Greek yogurt topped with 1/4 cup raspberries and 1 1/2 Tbsp. chopped walnuts

A.M. Snack (101 calories)

- 1 medium pear

Lunch (371 calories)

- 1 serving SlowCooker Turkey Chili with Butternut Squash
- 1 medium apple

P.M. Snack (35 calories)

- 1 clementine

Dinner (453 calories)

- 1 serving Polenta Bowls with Roasted Vegetables & Fried Eggs

Daily Totals: 1,213 calories, 69 g protein, 154 g carbohydrate, 31 g fiber, 41 g fat, 1,492 mg sodium

To make it 1,500 calories: Add 1/3 cup unsalted almonds to A.M. snack.

To make it 2,000 calories: Include the modification for the 1,500calorie day, plus increase to 1/4 cup walnuts and 1 1/4 cups yogurt at breakfast and add 2 slices wholewheat toast with 2 Tbsp. natural peanut butter to P.M. snack.

Week 2

How to MealPrep Your Week of Meals:

1. Prepare Mini Quiches with Sweet Potato Crust to have for breakfast on Days 9, 10 and 12. Freeze the remaining servings to have in Week 4.
2. Prepare Indian Grain Bowls with Chicken & Vegetables to have for lunch on Days 9 through 12.

Day 8

Breakfast (297 calories)

- 1 serving Pineapple Green Smoothie

A.M. Snack (101 calories)

- 1 medium pear

Lunch (360 calories)

- 1 serving White Bean & Veggie Salad

P.M. Snack (77 calories)

- 1 small apple

Dinner (374 calories)

- 1 serving Salmon & Asparagus with LemonGarlic Butter Sauce
- 1 serving Basic Quinoa

Daily Totals: 1,210 calories, 53 g protein, 156 g carbohydrate, 37 g fiber, 49 g fat, 824 mg sodium

To make it 1,500 calories: Add 1 clementine to breakfast and add 1/3 cup unsalted almonds to P.M. snack.

To make it 2,000 calories: Include all modifications for the 1,500calorie day, plus add 2 slices wholewheat toast with natural peanut butter to breakfast and add 1/4 cup walnuts to A.M. snack.

Day 9

Breakfast (251 calories)

- 1 serving Mini Quiches with Sweet Potato Crust
- 1 clementine

A.M. Snack (197 calories)

- 1 large pear
- 5 walnut halves

Lunch (297 calories)

- 1 serving Indian Grain Bowls with Chicken & Vegetables

P.M. Snack (62 calories)

- 1 medium orange

Dinner (390 calories)

- 1 serving FlatBelly Salad

Daily Totals: 1,197 calories, 61 g protein, 131 g carbohydrate, 32 g fiber, 52 g fat, 1,582 mg sodium

To make it 1,500 calories: Add 1/3 cup unsalted almonds to A.M. snack.

To make it 2,000 calories: Include the modification for the 1,500calorie day, plus add 1/4 cup walnuts to breakfast and add 2 slices wholewheat toast with 2 Tbsp. natural peanut butter to P.M. snack.

Day 10

Breakfast (251 calories)

- 1 serving Mini Quiches with Sweet Potato Crust
- 1 clementine

A.M. Snack (131 calories)

- 1 large pear

Lunch (332 calories)

- 1 serving Indian Grain Bowls with Chicken & Vegetables
- 1 clementine

P.M. Snack (116 calories)

- 1 large apple

Dinner (362 calories, 8 g fiber)

- 1 serving Chickpea Curry
- 1/2 (6inch) wholewheat pita bread

Daily Totals: 1,192 calories, 55 g protein, 173 g carbohydrate, 31 g fiber, 37 g fat, 1,448 mg sodium

To make it 1,500 calories: Add 1/3 cup unsalted almonds to A.M. snack.

To make it 2,000 calories: Include the modification for the 1,500calorie day, plus increase to 2 clementines at breakfast, add 1 serving Everything Bagel Avocado Toast to lunch, and add 3 Tbsp. natural peanut butter to P.M. snack.

Day 11

Breakfast (297 calories)

- 1 serving Pineapple Green Smoothie

A.M. Snack (131 calories)

- 1 large pear

Lunch (332 calories)

- 1 serving Indian Grain Bowls with Chicken & Vegetables
- 1 clementine

P.M. Snack (77 calories)

- – 1 small apple

Dinner (366 calories)

- – 1 serving Vegetarian Niçoise Salad

Daily Totals: 1,204 calories, 57 g protein, 175 g carbohydrate, 34 g fiber, 36 g fat, 1,251 mg sodium

To make it 1,500 calories: Add 1 medium orange to lunch and add 2 Tbsp. natural peanut butter to P.M. snack.

To make it 2,000 calories: Include all modifications for the 1,500calorie day, plus add 1 medium apple to breakfast, add 1/3 cup unsalted almonds to A.M. snack, and add 1/2 an avocado to dinner.

Day 12

MealPrep Tip: Prep the SlowCooker Vegetable Stew in the morning; set the slow cooker to Low and cook for 8 hours so it's ready in time for dinner.

Breakfast (251 calories)

- 1 serving Mini Quiches with Sweet Potato Crust
- 1 clementine

A.M. Snack (131 calories)

- 1 large pear

Lunch (332 calories)

- 1 serving Indian Grain Bowls with Chicken & Vegetables
- 1 clementine

P.M. Snack (77 calories)

- 1 small apple

Dinner (407 calories)

- 1 serving SlowCooker Vegetable Stew

MealPrep Tip: Reserve 2 servings SlowCooker Vegetable Stew to have for lunch on Days 13 and 14.

Daily Totals: 1,198 calories, 62 g protein, 177 g carbohydrate, 33 g fiber, 31 g fat, 1,754 mg sodium

To make it 1,500 calories: Add 1 medium orange to lunch and add 2 Tbsp. natural peanut butter to P.M. snack.

To make it 2,000 calories: Include all modifications for the 1,500calorie day, plus add 1 slice wholewheat toast with 1 Tbsp. natural peanut butter and 1 small apple to breakfast, and add 1/3 cup unsalted almonds to A.M. snack.

Day 13

Breakfast (287 calories)

- 1 serving Muesli with Raspberries

A.M. Snack (8 calories)

- 1/2 cup sliced cucumber tossed with a pinch each of salt & pepper

Lunch (407 calories)

- 1 serving SlwCooker Vegetable Stew

P.M. Snack (23 calories)

- 1 small bell pepper, sliced

Dinner (497 calories)

- 1 serving Spaghetti Squash & Chicken with Avocado Pesto

Daily Totals: 1,222 calories, 60 g protein, 147 g carbohydrate, 36 g fiber, 50 g fat, 1,603 mg sodium

To make it 1,500 calories: Add 1 medium apple to breakfast, add 3 Tbsp. hummus to A.M. snack, and add 1/4 cup guacamole to P.M. snack.

To make it 2,000 calories: Include all modifications for the 1,500calorie day, plus add 1 slice wholewheat toast with 1 Tbsp. natural peanut butter to breakfast, add 1/3 cup unsalted almonds to A.M. snack, and add 1 clementine to lunch.

Day 14

Breakfast (287 calories)

- 1 serving Muesli with Raspberries

A.M. Snack (62 calories)

- 1 medium orange

Lunch (407 calories)

- 1 serving SlowCooker Vegetable Stew

P.M. Snack (35 calories)

- 1 clementine

Dinner (429 calories)

- 1 serving Charred Shrimp & Pesto Buddha Bowls

Daily Totals: 1,220 calories, 62 g protein, 168 g carbohydrate, 37 g fiber, 40 g fat, 1,483 mg sodium

To make it 1,500 calories: Add 1/3 cup unsalted almonds to A.M. snack.

To make it 2,000 calories: Include all modifications for the 1,500calorie day, plus add 1 cup lowfat plain Greek yogurt and 2 slices wholewheat toast with 2 Tbsp. natural peanut butter to P.M. snack. 1 serving Chicken, Quinoa & Sweet Potato Casserole

Daily Totals: 1,185 calories, 61 g protein, 168 g carbohydrate, 31 g fiber, 34 g fat, 1,043 mg sodium

To make it 1,500 calories: Increase to 1/4 cup slivered almonds at breakfast and add 1/4 cup walnuts to P.M. snack.

To make it 2,000 calories: Include all modifications for the 1,500calorie day, plus add 3 Tbsp. unsalted almonds to A.M. snack and increase to 2 servings Chicken, Quinoa & Sweet Potato Casserole at dinner.

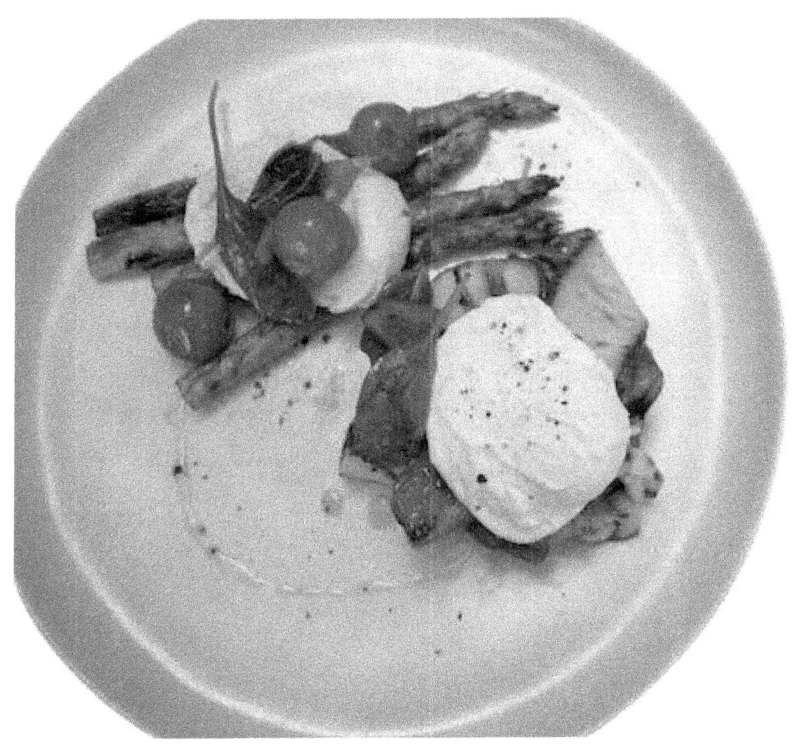

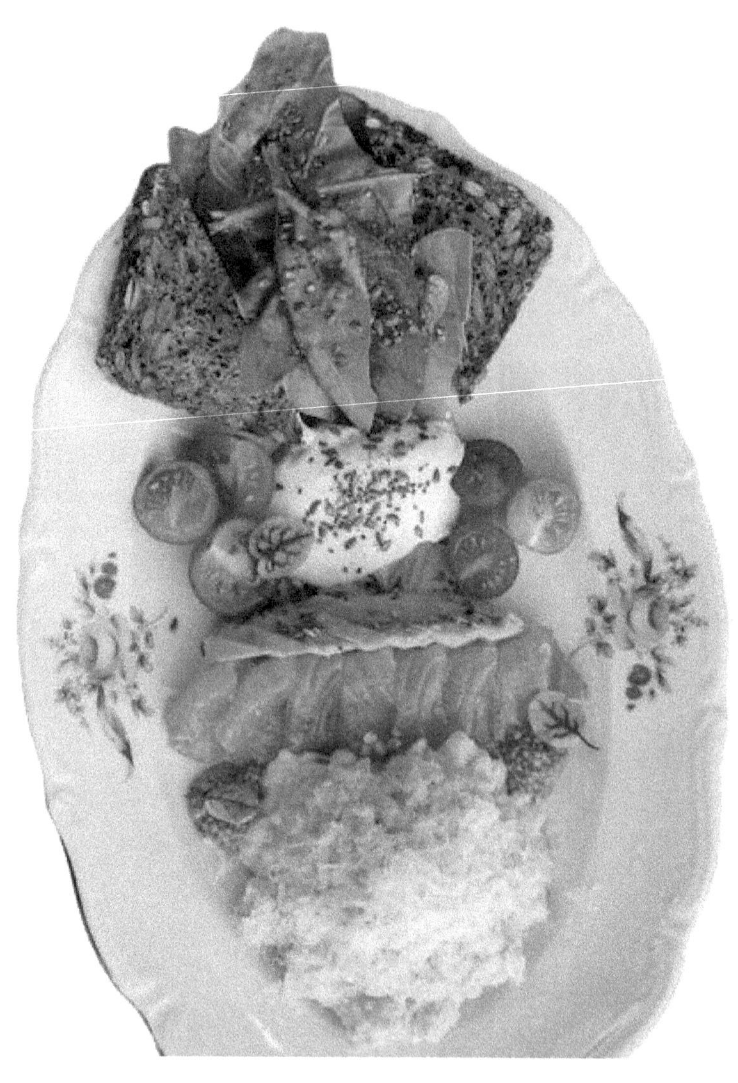

CHAPTER FOUR

Flat Stomach After Giving Birth Recipes

1. Individual Egg and Spinach Bowls

INGREDIENTS

- 8 egg whites large, recommend freerange
- 1 whole egg
- 1 cup baby spinach torn or chopped into small pieces
- 1/2 cup diced tomatoes
- 1/4 cup feta cheese fatfree
- 1/2 teaspoon black pepper
- kosher or sea salt to taste

INSTRUCTIONS

1. Preheat oven to 350 degrees.

2. Whisk together all ingredients in a medium mixing bowl. Lightly mist 4 (1/2 cup) ramekins with nonstick cooking spray and evenly divide egg mixture into bowls.

3. Place ramekins on a cookie sheet and bake 20 minutes or until eggs puff and are almost set in the center. Serve hot.

2. Avocado Egg Salad Sandwich

Double the flavor and nutrients with this new version of the egg salad sandwich that is quick and easy to make with only four ingredients.

INGREDIENTS

- 1/2 avocado ripe, pitted and peeled
- 1 boiled egg peeled and chopped
- 1/2 lemon freshly squeezed
- pinch kosher or sea salt
- 2 slices multigrain bread toasted if desired

INSTRUCTIONS

1. With a fork, mash the avocado, chopped boiled egg, lemon juice, and salt together just until combined. Overmixing will create an odd color, so you just want to mix until all ingredients are folded together.

2. Serve between two slices of multigrain bread. Enjoy!

3. Egg & Spinach Bell Pepper Bowls

You can even enjoy them as breakfast for dinner. Dig in and enjoy!

INGREDIENTS

- 2 eggs beaten
- 4 tablespoons feta cheese crumbled
- 1/2 teaspoon ground black pepper
- 1/4 teaspoon kosher salt
- 1/2 cup spinach cooked, and liquid squeezed out
- 1 red bell pepper cut in half, seeds removed

INSTRUCTIONS

1. Preheat oven to 350 degrees. Spray a baking sheet with nonstick spray.

2. Place the pepper halves onto the baking sheet, cut side up. Divide the cooked spinach and feta between the two halves. Pour eggs over top and sprinkle with salt and pepper.

3. Bake 15 to 20 minutes or until puffed and set. Let rest about 5to 10 minutes before serving.

4. Banana Walnut Overnight Oatmeal

INGREDIENTS

Oats

- 1/3 cup rolled oats
- 1/2 cup milk lowfat
- 1/3 cup yogurt plain, lowfat
- 1 tablespoon honey
- 1/4 teaspoon ground cinnamon
- 1/4 teaspoon vanilla extract
- pinch sea salt

For Serving

- 1/4 cup walnuts chopped
- 1 banana peeled and sliced

INSTRUCTIONS

1. Add all of the ingredients to two bowls or jars, cover, and stir to combine. Refrigerate for 68 hours.
2. When ready to serve, heat the oats in the microwave or enjoy chilled.
3. Top with the walnuts and banana slices just before serving.

5. Avocado Hummus Bowl

Give your body a boost of nutrients and energy with this amazing and delicious snack bowl.

INGREDIENTS

- 1/2 avocado ripe, peeled, pitted, and thickly sliced
- 1/2 cup chickpeas canned, drained and rinsed
- 1/2 cucumber medium, thinly sliced
- 2/3 cup grape tomatoes or cherry tomatoes
- 1 cup baby carrots
- 10 spinach leaves well cleaned
- 1/3 cup hummus clean eating, any variety, store bought or homemade
- 2 tablespoons pumpkin or shelled sunflower seeds, optional
- 1/4 teaspoon kosher or sea salt
- 1/4 teaspoon black pepper

INSTRUCTIONS

1. Line a bowl with spinach leaves, layering if necessary.
2. Add avocado slices to one corner, chickpeas to another, grape tomatoes to another, and baby carrots to another.

3. Add hummus to the center and top with sunflower or pumpkin seeds, if using.

4. Sprinkle whole dish with salt and pepper and enjoy!

5. This is great for a togo lunch when made in a portable container with a lid.

6. Grilled Turkey Burgers with Cucumber Salad

INGREDIENTS

Turkey Burgers

- 1 pound lean ground turkey

- 1 egg large, beaten

- 1/2 cup wholewheat breadcrumbs or wholewheat panko, plain

- 1/3 cup onions grated or finely chopped

- 1/3 cup parsley finely chopped

- 1 garlic clove minced

- 1/2 teaspoon kosher or sea salt

- 1/2 teaspoon black pepper

- 1 tablespoon extra virgin olive oil

- 2 teaspoons canola oil or cooking spray to lightly coat the pan or grill

Cucumber Salad

- 1 cucumber diced small

- 1/2 cup chives or green onions, chopped

- 1 tomato medium, ripe and finely diced

- 2 tablespoons lime juice or lemon juice, freshly squeezed

- 1/4 teaspoon kosher or sea salt

INTRUCTIONS

1. Combine all ingredients for turkey burgers, except olive oil.

2. Form into 4 to 5 patties.

3. Sprinkle each patty on both sides with olive oil, using fingers to coat. Lightly oil grates of grill.

4. Set grill to mediumhigh heat or place a lightlyoiled skillet or grill pan on the stovetop over mediumhigh heat.

5. Add patties to grill or skillet and cover (cover if using the grill) and grill for 5 to 6 minutes on each side, until cooked through.

6. Meanwhile, mix together all ingredients for cucumber salad. Serve room temperature or chill until serving.

7. Red PepperScallion Corn Muffin

The dash of spices in these corn muffins makes them a snack

or breakfast that packs a punch.

INGREDIENTS

- 2 Tbsp + 1/4 c canola oil, divided
- 1 large red bell pepper, coarsely chopped
- 4 scallions, thinly sliced
- 1½ c yellow cornmeal
- 1/2 c whole grain
- pastry flour
- 1¾ tsp baking powder
- 1/2 tsp salt
- 1/4 tsp baking soda
- 1/8 tsp freshly ground black pepper
- 1 c fatfree plain yogurt
- large egg
- large egg whites 2 tsp brown sugar
- 3/4 c drained canned vacuumpacked corn kernels (about 1/2 an 11ounce can)

INSTRUCTIONS

1. PREHEAT oven to 350°F. Coat Texassize, 6cup muffin tin with cooking spray or line with paper baking cups.

2. WARM 2 Tbsp of the oil in medium skillet over medium heat. Add bell pepper and cook, stirring, 5 minutes or until tender. Add scallions. Cook, stirring, 1 minute or until softened. Remove from heat and let cool 5 minutes.

3. STIR together cornmeal, flour, baking powder, salt, baking soda, and black pepper in large bowl. In medium bowl, whisk together yogurt, egg, egg whites, sugar, and remaining 1/4 c oil. Fold in bell pepper mixture and corn. Fold into dry ingredients until just moistened.

4. DIVIDE batter evenly among prepared muffin cups. Bake 25 to 30 minutes or until wooden pick inserted in center comes out clean. Cool in pan on wire rack 5 minutes. Remove muffins from pan to cool completely on wire rack.

8. Hearty Roast Beef Panini

TIME: 10 minutes

SERVINGS: 1

- 2 slices reducedcalorie multigrain bread
- 2 ounces storeroasted, delisliced lean roast beef
- 2 beefsteak tomato slices
- 1/4 avocado, sliced
- 1/8 cup baby arugula
- 1 tsp Dijon mustard
- 1/4 tsp extra virgin olive oil

INSTRUCTIONS

1. PLACE 1 slice of the bread on a work surface. Top with the roast beef, tomato slices, avocado slices, and arugula. Spread the remaining bread with mustard and set, mustard side down, on the arugula.

2. HEAT a ridged nonstick grill pan over medium heat until hot. Lightly brush the outsides of the sandwich with the oil and place on the pan. Set a heavybottomed skillet on top of the sandwich and cook for 1 to 2 minutes per side or until toasted and warm in the center.

9. Turkey Meat Loaf with Walnuts and Sage

What could be better than a comfortfood recipe with belly slimming benefits? Walnuts and whole wheat breadcrumbs pack this classicwithatwist dish with fiber and a nutty taste.

INGREDIENTS

- 2 tsp olive oil
- 1 large carrot, grated
- 4 scallions, thinly sliced
- 1 clove garlic, minced
- 1/2 cup walnuts (MUFA) 2
- slices whole wheat bread
- 1/4 cup fatfree milk
- egg whites, lightly beaten
- 1pound extralean ground turkey breast (99% fatfree)
- 1/4 cup chopped fresh flatleaf parsley
- 1/4 cup grated Parmesan cheese
- 1 tsp dried sage
- 1/2 tsp salt
- 1/2 tsp freshly ground black pepper

INSTRUCTIONS

1. PREHEAT the oven to 350°F. Line a rimmed baking sheet with foil and coat the foil with olive oil spray.

2. HEAT the oil in a small nonstick skillet over medium heat. Add the carrot, scallions, and garlic and cook, stirring often, for about 3 minutes or until tender. Remove from the heat.

3. MEANWHILE, chop the walnuts in a food processor fitted with a metal blade. Break up the bread and add to the walnuts. Pulse until both are ground to fine crumbs. Transfer to a large bowl. With a fork, stir in the milk and egg whites. Add the turkey, parsley, cheese, sage, salt, pepper, and sautéed mixture. Mix gently just until blended.

4. SHAPE into a freeform loaf about 7" long and 4 1/2" wide on the prepared baking sheet. Bake for 50 to 60 minutes or until a thermometer inserted in the thickest portion registers 165°F. Let stand a few minutes before slicing.

10. Slow Cooker Moroccan Chicken with Olives

Minimize your kitchen time with this slowcooked ethnic soup. If you like spicy food use a hotter pepper, such as chile de arbol, instead of the milder guajillo.

INGREDIENTS

Chicken

- 1/2 cup reducedsodium chicken broth
- 1/4 cup allpurpose flour
- Tbsp olive oil
- 2 tsp ground cumin
- 1/2 tsp freshly ground black pepper
- 1/4 tsp salt
- 1 can (14½ ounces) nosaltadded stewed tomatoes 1 carrot, sliced
- 1 large onion
- 30 small black olives, pitted (about 1 cup)
- 3 cloves garlic, minced
- 2 pounds boneless, skinless chicken breast halves
- 1/2 cup chopped fresh cilantro (optional)

Harissa

- 3/4 cup dried hot red chile peppers, such as guajillo
- 2 cloves garlic, minced
- 1 tsp ground coriander
- 1 tsp ground caraway seed
- 1/4 tsp salt
- 3 Tbsp olive oil

INSTRUCTIONS

1. PREPARE the chicken: Coat the stoneware of a slow cooker pot with cooking spray.
2. Combine the broth, flour, oil, cumin, pepper, and salt in the pot.
3. Whisk until smooth. Add the tomatoes (with juice), carrot, onion, olives, and garlic.
4. Stir to mix. Tuck the chicken into the pot, covering with the other ingredients. Cover and cook on low for 5 to 6 hours or on high for 3 to 4 hours.
5. PREPARE the harissa: Remove the stems and seeds from the peppers and discard. Soak the peppers in warm water for about 1 hour or until softened.
6. Drain and transfer to a food processor fitted with a metal blade or a blender.

7. Add the garlic, coriander, caraway seed, and salt.

8. Process, scraping the sides of the bowl as needed, until a paste forms. Drizzle in the oil through the tube to reach a smooth consistency.

9. STIR in the cilantro (if using) just before serving. Pass the harissa at the table.

11. Chicken Piccata

This Italianstyle dish is packed with protein and sure to please any palate.

Whip up this lemonchicken recipe any weeknight for a simple—slimming—evening meal.

INGREDIENTS

- 12 ounces boneless, skinless chicken tenders
- 2 Tbsp flour
- 4 Tbsp olive oil
- 2 freshly squeezed lemon juice
- 2 Tbsp chopped fresh parsley
- 2 tsp capers, minced
- Freshly ground black pepper

INSTRUCTIONS

1. LAY the tenders on a work surface. With a smooth scaloppine pounder or a rolling pin covered in plastic wrap, flatten to 1/4" thickness. Dredge the cutlets lightly in the flour.

2. HEAT a large skillet over mediumhigh heat. Add the oil to the skillet and heat until sizzling. Place the chicken in the skillet. Cook for 2 minutes per side or until lightly browned and cooked through.

3. ADD the lemon juice, parsley, and capers. Bring the mixture to a boil. Reduce the heat and simmer for 2 minutes to allow the flavors to blend. Season to taste with the pepper. Serve the chicken with the pan juices.

1. Note: Pounding the chicken breasts to an even thickness is an important step because it allows the chicken to cook evenly so both ends are moist and delicious.

12. Slow Cooker African Chicken Stew

Prep this stew in the morning and come home to a fragrant, onepot dinner. The chicken, carrots, and potatoes in this hearty stew are sure to leave you feeling satisfied.

As much as possible, avoid the temptation to lift the lid when using a slow cooker. Every time you take a peek, it takes 20 to 30 minutes for the cooking temperature to return to where it was.

INGREDIENTS

- 1 Tbsp peanut oil
- 12 ounces boneless, skinless chicken thighs, trimmed and cut into 24 pieces
- 1 onion, chopped
- 3 cloves garlic, minced
- 1 jalapeno chile pepper, seeded and chopped
- 1 carrot, thickly sliced
- sweet potato, peeled and cubed
- can (14½ ounces) reduced sodium chicken broth
- 1/2 cup chunky natural unsalted peanut butter
- Tbsp tomato paste
- 1/4 tsp salt
- 1/4 tsp freshly ground black pepper

INSTRUCTIONS

1. HEAT the oil in a large nonstick skillet over mediumhigh heat. Add the chicken and cook, stirring occasionally, for 3 to 4 minutes or until lightly browned.
2. Transfer to a 4quart slow cooker. Return the skillet to the heat and add the onion, garlic, chile pepper, and carrot.
3. Cook for 1 minute, then transfer to the slow cooker.
4. Stir in the sweet potato, broth, peanut butter, and tomato paste.
5. COOK on high for 3 to 4 hours or low for 5 to 6 hours or until the chicken and vegetables are very tender. Season with salt and black pepper.

13. Greek Yogurt Parfait

INGREDIENTS

- 1 cup Greek yogurt
- 1/2 cup mixed berries (blueberries, strawberries, raspberries)
- 2 tablespoons chopped nuts (e.g., almonds or walnuts)
- 1 tablespoon honey

Method

1. In a glass or bowl, layer Greek yogurt, mixed berries, and chopped nuts.
2. Drizzle with honey and serve.

14. Oatmeal with Nut Butter and Banana

INGREDIENTS:

- 1/2 cup old fashioned oats
- 1 cup milk (of your choice)
- 1 tablespoon nut butter (e.g., almond or peanut)
- 1 banana, sliced
- 1 teaspoon honey
- Cinnamon (optional)

Method:

1. Cook oats according to package instructions in milk.
2. Top with sliced banana, nut butter, honey, and a sprinkle of cinnamon if desired.

15. Grilled Chicken and Quinoa Bowl

INGREDIENTS:

- 2 boneless, skinless chicken breasts
- 2 cups cooked quinoa
- 1 cup steamed broccoli

- 1/2 cup sliced bell peppers

- 1/4 cup sliced avocado

- Olive oil

- Lemon juice

- Salt and pepper to taste

Method:

1. Preheat the grill to mediumhigh heat.

2. Season the chicken breasts with olive oil, lemon juice, salt, and pepper.

3. Grill the chicken for about 67 minutes per side until cooked through.

4. Slice the chicken into strips.

5. In a bowl, combine cooked quinoa, steamed broccoli, sliced bell peppers, and avocado.Top with grilled chicken strips and serve.

16. Salmon and Asparagus

INGREDIENTS:

- 2 salmon fillets

- 1 bunch of asparagus spears

- Olive oil

- Lemon slices

- Salt and pepper to taste

Method:

1. Preheat the oven to 375°F (190°C).

2. Place asparagus spears on a baking sheet, drizzle with olive oil, and season with salt and pepper. Roast for about 1520 minutes.

3. Season the salmon fillets with olive oil, lemon slices, salt, and pepper.

4. Bake the salmon in the same oven for about 1520 minutes or until cooked through.

5. Serve the salmon on a bed of roasted asparagus.

17. Quinoa and Black Bean Salad

INGREDIENTS:

- 1 cup quinoa
- 1 can black beans, drained and rinsed
- 1 cup diced tomatoes
- 1 cup diced cucumbers
- 1/2 cup chopped fresh cilantro
- Juice of 1 lime
- 2 tablespoons olive oil
- Salt and pepper to taste

Method:

1. Cook quinoa according to package instructions and let it cool.

2. In a large bowl, combine quinoa, black beans, tomatoes, cucumbers, and cilantro.

3. In a small bowl, whisk together lime juice, olive oil, salt, and pepper.

4. Drizzle the dressing over the salad and toss to combine.

18. Lentil and Vegetable Soup

INGREDIENTS:

- 1 cup dried lentils, rinsed and drained
- 2 carrots, chopped
- 2 celery stalks, chopped
- 1 onion, chopped
- 2 cloves garlic, minced
- 6 cups vegetable or chicken broth
- 1 bay leaf
- 1 teaspoon dried thyme
- Salt and pepper to taste

Method:

1. In a large pot, sauté onions, garlic, carrots, and celery in a bit of olive oil until they begin to soften.
2. Add lentils, vegetable or chicken broth, bay leaf, and thyme to the pot. Bring to a boil.
3. Reduce heat, cover, and simmer for 2530 minutes or until lentils and vegetables are tender.
4. Remove the bay leaf and season with salt and pepper.
5. Serve hot.

19. Egg and Vegetable Omelette

INGREDIENTS:

- 2 eggs
- 1/2 cup diced bell peppers (any color)
- 1/4 cup diced onions
- 1/4 cup diced tomatoes
- 1/4 cup grated cheese (optional)
- Olive oil
- Salt and pepper to taste

Method:

1. In a bowl, beat the eggs and season with salt and pepper.

2. Heat a nonstick skillet over medium heat with a bit of olive oil.

3. Add onions, bell peppers, and tomatoes to the skillet and sauté for a few minutes until slightly softened.

4. Pour the beaten eggs over the vegetables and cook until set.

5. If desired, sprinkle grated cheese over half of the omelette and fold it in half.

6. Serve hot.

20. Vegetable and Chickpea Curry

INGREDIENTS:

- 1 can chickpeas, drained and rinsed

- 1 cup chopped cauliflower

- 1 cup chopped broccoli

- 1 cup chopped carrots

- 1 onion, chopped

- 2 cloves garlic, minced

- 1 can diced tomatoes

- 1 can coconut milk

- 2 tablespoons curry powder
- Salt and pepper to taste
- Cooked brown rice

Method:

1. In a large pot, sauté onions, garlic, carrots, and celery in a bit of olive oil until they begin to soften.
2. Add the curry powder and cook for another minute.
3. Add the chickpeas, cauliflower, broccoli, carrots, diced tomatoes, and coconut milk. Bring to a simmer and cook for 2025 minutes or until the vegetables are tender.
4. Season with salt and pepper.
5. Serve over cooked brown rice.

21. Healthy Turkey and Vegetable StirFry

INGREDIENTS:

- 1 pound ground turkey
- 2 cups broccoli florets
- 1 red bell pepper, sliced
- 1 cup snap peas, trimmed
- 2 cloves garlic, minced
- 1/4 cup lowsodium soy sauce
- 2 tablespoons hoisin sauce

- 1 tablespoon olive oil

- Cooked brown rice

Method:

1. In a small bowl, whisk together soy sauce and hoisin sauce to make the sauce.

2. Heat a large skillet or wok over high heat with olive oil.

3. Add ground turkey and cook until browned and cooked through.

4. Remove the cooked turkey from the skillet.

5. In the same skillet, add broccoli, red bell pepper, snap peas, and garlic. Stirfry for about 45 minutes until vegetables are tendercrisp.

6. Return the cooked turkey to the skillet, pour the sauce over everything, and cook for another 2 minutes.

7. Serve over cooked brown rice.

22. Baked Sweet Potato with Cottage Cheese

INGREDIENTS:

- 1 large sweet potato

- 1/2 cup lowfat cottage cheese

- 1/4 cup copped fresh chives

- Salt and pepper to taste

Method:

1. Preheat the oven to 375°F (190°C).

2. Pierce the sweet potato with a fork a few times and place it on a baking sheet.

3. Bake for about 4560 minutes or until the sweet potato is tender when pierced with a fork.

4. Split the sweet potato open and fluff the inside with a fork.

5. Top with cottage cheese, chopped chives, salt, and pepper

23. Salmon Salad with Avocado and Greens

INGREDIENTS:

- 2 salmon fillets
- Mixed greens (e.g., spinach, arugula
- 1 avocado, sliced
- Cherry tomatoes, halved
- Olive oil
- Balsamic vinegar
- Salt and pepper to taste

Method:

1. Season salmon fillets with olive oil, salt, and pepper. Gril or bake until cooked through.
2. In a bowl, toss mixed greens with a drizzle of olive oil and balsamic vinegar.
3. Top greens with grilled salmon, avocado slices, and cherry tomatoes.
4. Season with additional salt and pepper if desired.

24. Mango and Quinoa Salad

Ingredients:

- 1 cup cooked quinoa
- 1 ripe mango, diced
- 1/2 cucumber, diced
- 1/4 cup red onion, finely chopped
- Fresh cilantro, chopped
- Lime juice
- Olive oil
- Salt and pepper to taste

Method:

1. In a bowl, combine cooked quinoa, diced mango, diced cucumber, and chopped red onion.

2. Drizzle with lime juice and olive oil.

3. Add fresh cilantro for flavor.

4. Season with salt and pepper to taste.

25. Lentil and Vegetable StirFry

Ingredients:

- 1 cup cooked lentils

- Mixed vegetables (e.g., bell peppers, snap peas, carrots), sliced

- 2 cloves garlic, minced

- Ginger, grated

- Lowsodium soy sauce

- Sesame oil

- Cooked brown rice

Method:

1. Heat a skillet or wok over high heat with a bit of sesame oil.

2. Add minced garlic and grated ginger, stirfry for a minute.

3. Add mixed vegetables and cook until tendercrisp.

4. Stir in cooked lentils and a splash of lowsodium soy sauce.

5. Serve over cooked brown rice.

26. Stuffed Bell Peppers

INGREDIENTS:

- Bell peppers (any color), halved and cleaned
- Lean ground turkey or chicken
- Cooked quinoa
- Chopped tomatoes
- Onion, finely chopped
- Garlic, minced
- Olive oil
- Italian seasoning
- Salt and pepper to taste

Method:

1. Preheat the oven to 375°F (190°C)

2. In a skillet, sauté chopped onion and minced garlic in olive oil.

3. Add ground turkey or chicken and cook until browned.

4. Stir in cooked quinoa, chopped tomatoes, and Italian seasoning.

5. Fill bell pepper halves with the mixture.

6. Place stuffed peppers in a baking dish, cover with foil, and bake for about 3035 minutes or until peppers are tender.

27. Chia Seed Pudding with Berries

INGREDIENTS:

- 2 tablespoons chia seeds
- 1 cup milk (of your choice)
- 1/2 teaspoon vanilla extract
- Mixed berries (e.g., strawberries, blueberries, raspberries)

Method:

1. In a bowl, combine chia seeds, milk, and vanilla extract.

2. Stir well and refrigerate for at least 2 hours or until it thickens.

3. Serve with mixed berries on top.

28. Turkey and Vegetable Soup

INGREDIENTS:

- Lean ground turkey
- Mixed vegetables (e.g., carrots, celery, zucchini), chopped

- Lowsodium chicken broth
- Onion, finely chopped
- Garlic, minced
- Olive oil
- Fresh herbs (e.g., thyme, rosemary)
- Salt and pepper to taste

Method:

1. In a large pot, sauté chopped onion and minced garlic in olive oil.
2. Add ground turkey and cook until browned.
3. Add chopped vegetables, fresh herbs, and lowsodium chicken broth.
4. Simmer until the vegetables are tender.
5. Season with salt and pepper to taste.

29. Healthy Berry Smoothie

INGREDIENTS:

- 1 cup mixed berries (e.g., strawberries, blueberries, raspberries)
- 1/2 cup Greek yogurt
- 1/2 cup spinach (for added nutrients)
- 1/2 cup milk (of your choice)
- 1 tablespoon honey

Method:

1. Blend all ingredients in a blender until smooth.

2. Adjust the consistency by adding more milk if needed.

3. Serve immediately.

30. Quinoa and Chickpea Salad

INGREDIENTS:

- 1 cup cooked quinoa

- 1 can chickpeas, drained and rinsed

- Cherry tomatoes, halved

- Cucumber, diced

- Red onion, finely chopped

- Fresh parsley, chopped

- Feta cheese (optional)

- Lemon vinaigrette dressing (olive oil, lemon juice, garlic, salt, and pepper)

Method:

1. In a large bowl, combine cooked quinoa, chickpeas, cherry tomatoes, cucumber, red onion, and fresh parsley.

2. If desired, add crumbled feta cheese for extra flavor

3. Drizzle with lemon vinaigrette dressing and toss to combine.

31. Baked Chicken and Vegetable Skewers

INGREDIENTS:

- Chicken breast, cut into chunks
- Bell peppers (various colors), sliced
- Red onion, cut into wedges
- Zucchini, sliced
- Cherry tomatoes
- Olive oil
- Garlic powder, paprika, salt, and pepper

Method:

1. Preheat the oven to 375°F (190°C) or use a grill.
2. Thread chicken and vegetables onto skewers.
3. Brush with olive oil and sprinkle with garlic powder, paprika, salt, and pepper.
4. Bake in the oven or grill until the chicken is cooked through and the vegetables are tender.

32. Spinach and Mushroom Stuffed Chicken Breast

INGREDIENTS:

- Boneless, skinless chicken breasts
- Fresh spinach leaves

- Sliced mushrooms

- Garlic, minced

- Olive oil

- Lowsodium chicken broth

- Salt and pepper to taste

Method:

1. Preheat the oven to 375°F (190°C).

2. In a skillet, sauté sliced mushrooms and minced garlic in olive oil until mushrooms are tender.

3. Butterfly the chicken breasts and stuff with fresh spinach leaves and the sautéed mushroom mixture.

4. Season with salt and pepper.

5. Bake in the oven until the chicken is cooked through.

33. Sweet Potato and Black Bean Tacos

INGREDIENTS:

- Sweet potatoes, diced

- Black beans, cooked and drained

- Red onion, finely chopped

- Cilantro, chopped

- Lime wedges

- Corn tortillas

- Olive oil

- Cumin, paprika, salt, and pepper

Method:

1. Preheat the oven to 375°F (190°C).

2. Toss diced sweet potatoes with olive oil, cumin, paprika, salt, and pepper.

3. Roast in the oven until tender and slightly crispy.

4. Warm corn tortillas.

5. Fill tortillas with roasted sweet potatoes, black beans, red onion, and cilantro.

6. Serve with lime wedges for squeezing.

34. Mediterranean Chickpea Salad

INGREDIENTS:

- 2 cans chickpeas, drained and rinsed

- Cucumber, diced

- Cherry tomatoes, halved

- Red onion, finely chopped

- Kalamata olives, pitted and sliced

- Feta cheese (optional)

- Fresh parsley, chopped

- Olive oil, lemon juice, garlic, salt, and pepper for dressing

Method:

1. In a large bowl, combine chickpeas, cucumber, cherry tomatoes, red onion, Kalamata olives, and fresh parsley.

2. If desired, add crumbled feta cheese.

3. Prepare a dressing with olive oil, lemon juice, minced garlic, salt, and pepper.

4. Drizzle the dressing over the salad and toss to combine.

35. Roasted Vegetable and Quinoa Bowl

INGREDIENTS:

- 1 cup cooked quinoa
- Mixed roasted vegetables (e.g., sweet potatoes, Brussels sprouts, cauliflower)
- Chickpeas, roasted
- Tahini dressing (tahini, lemon juice, garlic, salt, and pepper)

Method:

1. Toss mixed vegetables and chickpeas with olive oil, salt, and pepper.

2. Roast in the oven until tender and slightly caramelized.

3. Serve over cooked quinoa and drizzle with tahini dressing.

Flat Stomach Exercises After Pregnancy

Exercising after pregnancy can help you regain strength and tone your abdominal muscles.

Here are 10 flat stomach exercises after pregnancy and how to do them. Remember to consult with your healthcare provider before starting any postpregnancy exercise routine, especially if you've had a Csection or experienced any complications during childbirth.

1. Pelvic Tilts

How to do it:

1. Lie on your back with your knees bent and feet flat on the floor.

2. Inhale, then exhale as you tilt your pelvis upward, flattening your lower back against the floor.

3. Hold for a few seconds, then release.

4. Repeat for 1015 reps.

2. Kegel Exercises

How to do it:

1. Sit or lie down comfortably.
2. Tighten your pelvic floor muscles as if you're trying to stop the flow of urine.
3. Hold for a few seconds, then release.
4. Repcat this exercise for 1015 reps.

3. Leg Slides

How to do it:

1. Lie on your back with your knees bent and feet flat on the floor.
2. Slowly slide one leg out straight while keeping the other bent.
3. Hold for a few seconds, then return to the starting position.
4. Repeat with the other leg.
5. Do 1015 reps on each leg.

4. Bridge Pose

How to do it:

1. Lie on your back with your knees bent, feet hipwidth apart, and arms at your sides.

2. Inhale, then exhale as you lift your hips off the ground, creating a straight line from shoulders to knees.

3. Hold for a few seconds, then lower your hips.

4. Repeat for 1015 reps.

5. Diaphragmatic Breathing

How to do it:

1. Sit or lie down comfortably.

2. Place one hand on your chest and the other on your abdomen.

3. Inhale deeply through your nose, expanding your abdomen.

4. Exhale slowly through your mouth, allowing your abdomen to deflate.

5. Repeat for several breaths to engage your core muscles.

6. Planks

How to do it:

1. Start in a pushup position with your arms straight, or you can do a modified version on your forearms.

2. Keep your body in a straight line from head to heels.

3. Engage your core by pulling your navel toward your spine.

4. Hold for as long as you can, aiming for 30 seconds to 1 minute.

5. Repeat 23 times.

6. Modified PushUps

How to do it:

1. Start in a pushup position on your knees with your hands shoulderwidth apart.

2. Lower your chest toward the ground, keeping your body in a straight line.

3. Push back up to the starting position.

4. Repeat for 1015 reps.

7. Russian Twists

How to do it:

1. Sit on the floor with your knees bent and feet flat.

2. Lean back slightly and lift your feet off the ground, balancing on your sit bones.

3. Hold your hands together or use a weight or medicine ball.

4. Twist your torso to the right, then to the left, touching the object to the floor on each side.

5. Repeat for 1015 reps on each side.

8. Superman Exercise

How to do it:

1. Lie face down on the floor with your arms extended in front of you and your legs straight.
2. Lift your arms and legs off the ground as high as you can, engaging your lower back and glutes.
3. Hold for a few seconds, then lower back down.
4. Repeat for 1015 reps.

9. Side Planks

How to do it:

1. Lie on your side with your legs straight and your elbow directly beneath your shoulder.
2. Lift your hips off the ground, creating a straight line from head to heels.
3. Hold for as long as you can, aiming for 30 seconds to 1 minute.
4. Repeat on the other side.
5. Do 23 sets on each side.

Perform these exercises regularly, gradually increasing the intensity and duration as your strength and fitness levels improve.

CONCLUSION

You should aim to include two portions of vegetables, a portion of fruits, whole grains, and healthy protein. One of the most helpful tips for a flat tummy after pregnancy is to reduce your intake of salt and cut sugar out as much as you can. Avoid sodas and other carbonated drinks.

Cruciferous fruits and vegetables like papaya, mangoes, grapefruit, broccoli, and kale are great when it comes to losing abdominal fat.

In concluding "Flat Stomach After Pregnancy," we have embarked on a transformative journey that celebrates the resilience and strength of women during one of life's most profound phases.

Throughout the pages of this book, we've explored not just the physical aspect of reclaiming a toned midsection but also the emotional and mental dimensions of postpregnancy wellness.

This journey has revealed that achieving a flat stomach after pregnancy is more than just a physical goal; it's a testament to the power of determination, selfcare, and selfacceptance.

Yet, beyond the practical guidance, we've discovered a deeper truth—that the journey to a flat stomach is inseparable from the journey of motherhood itself.

It's a journey that encompasses selflove, selfcompassion, and the understanding that our bodies, having brought new life into the world, deserve our utmost care and respect.

As we close this book, let it serve as a source of empowerment and inspiration for every woman who has embarked on the path of postpregnancy transformation.

May it remind you that the journey towards a flat stomach is a testament to your strength, your commitment, and your enduring love for both yourself and your child.

Embrace this journey as an opportunity to rediscover the incredible strength within you and to celebrate the beauty of your evolving body.

May it be a journey filled with love, selfacceptance, and the unwavering belief that you are not just reclaiming your flat stomach; you are embracing the remarkable journey of motherhood itself, in all its glory and grace.

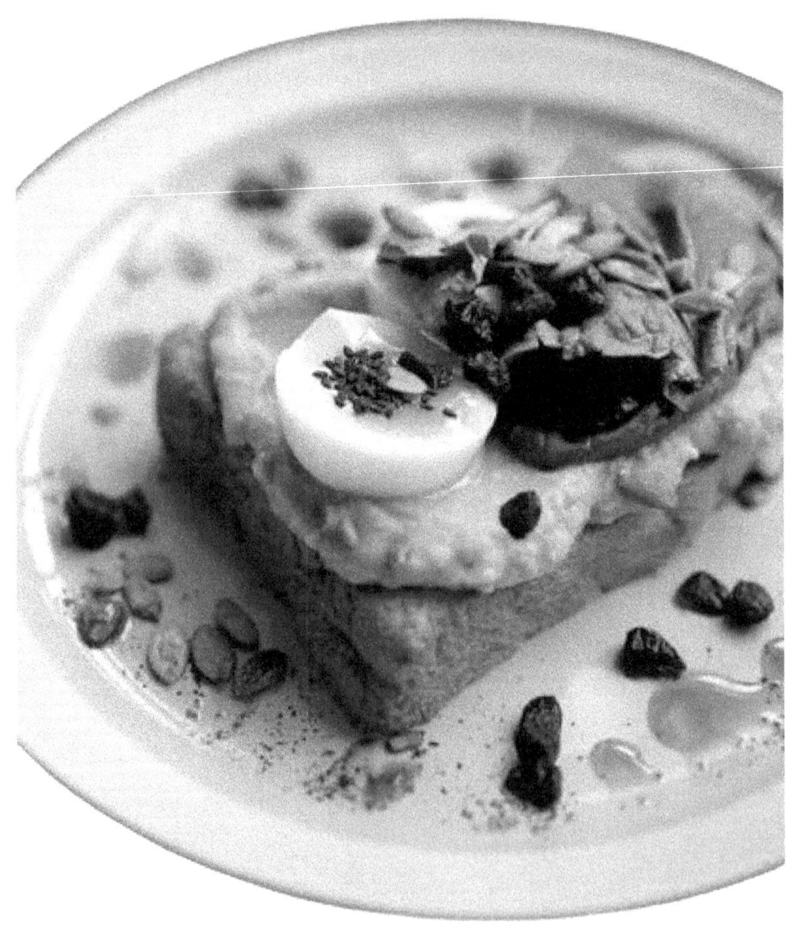